Epistle to
the Sisters
(and the brothers too)

Dr. C. P. Scott

DEDICATION

To every soul who has touched me even for a second.
You have contributed to who I am.

CONTENTS

ACKNOWLEDGMENTS

I want to acknowledge foremost God, the Father, Son, and Holy Spirit; my father Dr. Clarence Scott and my mothers Theodoris Bertha Scott and Dermerdine Shird Scott; my closest friend Shawni Richardson; every family member and friend who has shared stories, insights, opinions or support; each church and community group where I have been a part; the programs that have fed into my personal growth, with special thanks to Diazina Mobley, MSW, LCSW, of Mindful Guidance Solutions.

1 GREETINGS

With joy mixed with haste, I write to you. You see I've been wanting to reach out and share the happenings going on with me. Given what I know about you, you've been struggling with the same issues. You know we talked about it here and there—the lowest on the totem pool of humanity, the statistic, the dismissed, and the caricatures. The fact we have to claim and push forth our magic, instead of being valued and absorbed as an essential element of existence, is more than frustrating; it is suicide to creation.

That is strong language, but I believe with my heart that the world is imbalanced and on a downward spiral. The European masculine has dominated and ruled. All other aspects fall in line after and are allowed to move in, to operate in line with, this structure. Can you imagine? I speak and see the world with a Christian lens, which I find holds the complete essence of what it means to be human - in past, present and future. It is the most complete package of truth I have experienced. So I believe and will boldly hope that the scholars would agree the perfect and original plan is humans both masculine and feminine dominate together and not over one another with no arbitrary divisions of race and creed. We are just human beings, caretakers of one of the greatest gifts in the universe—the earth. What if Jesus was all about restoring balance? He was the spark to right the wheel, to tell us that we all in time are missing the point, missing the joy, missing the gist of this life. Hey, it is apparent that our masculine sides have a vested interest in not righting the ship even if it means we sink. Personally, I don't want to sink and I am pretty sure you don't want to either.

This is heavy stuff, but I want to start the conversation with you and shake us up a bit. I am in this with you and know that we can orchestrate an incredible coup, but not a coup to take over the ship. Even better in my mind, we use our magic to transform and evolve what we have into a totally different transportation. "For we know that the whole creation groaneth and travaileth in pain together until now." (Romans 8:22)

Humanity is a body with a disease ravaging its organism because it is not feeding and nurturing and honoring the majority of its members. It is like taking only the types of food to beef up one's testosterone and ignoring other nourishment. How would that work for a person, man or woman? You know what I read—too much testosterone causes infertility, non-production, non-multiplication whether in a male or a female. Human beings are meant to produce good in this earth, and not just other little human beings. We are to bear fruit, it is what we do. A fully functioning and engaged human being is magnificent in what she or he can create. We are the masterpiece of our Creator.   Take one minute! How ridiculous and awesome is that fact?! We were created to create; I want to sit in this sentence.

Well, you may wonder how I got to this "aha!" place. You can read the excitement I have. It is because I think I am getting it. Like, I think I am really getting this journey called life. Let me start from my awakening, because that moment was an explosion that shattered the rose-colored glasses, the delusions, and the chains on my mind. We haven't had a chance to really talk about that time about five years ago, but I am going to do so now because it is important context.

2 THE AWAKENING

On February 21, 2013, I confirmed with certainty that my fiancé was cheating on me. We had been together for fifteen months. He was in a parallel relationship for eight of those months. Of course there were suspicions and signs, I doubted and questioned the data I was receiving. Also, I wanted to believe the man I loved was honorable and would not lie to me about something so important. I wanted to believe that he would end our relationship before he would enter into another one.

What compounded the pain was that I accepted his proposal for marriage on the New Year's Eve that just past, even with red flags fluttering frantically inside of me. The day that I could no longer ignore the data without fully entering the realm of non-reality was the day that I communicated with the other woman who also was in the dark. The only difference between my relationship with him and her relationship with him was a ring. We together decided to cut our relationship with him immediately instead of risking a confrontation.

The cutting of the cords was critical for me. I was in trauma, ripped open and exposed. I was bleeding in front of everyone and I could not hide the pain. I had posted on Facebook the engagement. I had so many congratulations from church, work, friends, family. Now I went through the process of notifying and explaining and showing emotions I didn't ever want the external world to see in me. I shed tears in a professional meeting to tell my bosses that I needed to take some leave because of my broken engagement.

Weirdly, I felt relief and freedom because I knew the truth. During the relationship, my mind rode a rollercoaster of "am I crazy" "is he lying" "something is wrong" "I am being paranoid". Once I knew and accepted the truth, I came up to the surface for air and could breath. In not drowning and now conscious, I realized my humiliation and embarrassment. People could see me naked. Once your worst nightmare is no longer in your head and real and exposed, there is no room for pretending or trying to pretend. Because I had been drowning in a sea of lies for what seemed like eons, I would rather be alive and people see me then to have remained in that hell where death was certain, whether in body, soul, or both. Also, I saw looking in that sea, that some of those lies were mine.

My closest friend advised me to go into my place of prayer and lay on my face and turn to God. With intense pain, with gratefulness of an escape from a destructive path, with anger at feeling unprotected and unshielded from even experiencing such pain, with complete disappointment at life and God, I laid prostrate and cried out to God. I cried out all the emotions and fears and complaints and emptied myself. We are spiritual beings and to ignore this is a real detriment to our lives. When we access our spirit and allow communication with God, God answers always. I will get more into this later. While I was on my face, the lies and wayward thinking regarding my place in the world, regarding relationships with people and God, regarding my decisions, and regarding my worldview, sloughed off.

I experienced trauma—a deeply distressing or disturbing experience; synonyms include: injury, damage, a wound. Yet, I experienced trauma in a way I had not in the past. This post-trauma was not one of stress, in part due to the clean surgery of the situation. I experienced what I learned was post-traumatic growth. From the point I made the choice to not do a botched bandage job or pretend the wound did not exist which is the norm for me, I actually accelerated my healing. I allowed myself to let go and recognized that I did not have control and did not need control. If I made it and survived, it was because I submitted to the operating table to expose, clean and mend this gaping wound.

With any near-death experience, most of us want to move forward living our best life with greater appreciation for it. I entered a period where I wanted truth and more truth. I wanted to know truth even if I didn't like it. I wanted to live life to the max possibilities and I wanted to bring other women with me. I wanted to be exposed more and more so I would not slip into old mindsets and pretend. Reality is rich and richer than any make believe, with its highs and lows and in between, it holds treasure that is beyond the imagination.

Recovery is hard. Matter of fact, I am still healing although the scar is more faded. The scar is permanent. A healed scar is a sign of health and survival. My scar has been a springboard for connection with others especially women. It has been a ticket to entry on the path of personal growth and brought me closer to the abundant life promised in scripture—the land of being human, fully completely me.

3 THE REQUEST

A couple of months ago, I think I cracked the code, I found a map. It sat in plain sight the whole the time, but I could never figure it out. Maybe you already knew about this and figured it out, but please help me to review what I have and see if it is something. I am feeling acutely the struggle of women and especially women of color to be seen and heard and to be at the table of influence and decisions on humanity's direction. We are making strides yes; although it feels like for every two steps we take, the status quo takes five. If we don't figure out how to solve this imbalance in our world and get the majority to buy in, male or female, young or old, we dive to our extinction and the loss of the greatest gift of our universe. Eternity, other life, other worlds that may exist beyond our dimension will all grieve for the extinguished light of earth. The impact will be that of flap of a butterfly's wings. I do believe the majority of humanity will get it before it is too late, because I see awakenings happening in every corner with insight and wisdom flowing out of a myriad of springs. What I don't know is what healing will look like and how that will transform what we know, see and understand about this earth. The Bible speaks to this through Revelations, yet it is still beyond my ability to see a new earth, a new world.

The transformation of life as we know it begins as always with the basic unit of change, the individual. I want to review with you what has been gifted to me in knowledge and understanding on a personal level. It transformed my assumptions on which I based my choices which shape my emotions, my actions, and my position in life. If you agree and understand with me, I am confident it will lead to a tectonic shift for us as women, and especially women of color, for men, and for all, releasing our power, the expression of our true selves, and ultimately leading to what we envision—a balanced and thriving world where humanitarian isn't a niche population, it's the entire population.

4 SAFE SPACES

I guess the best way to approach this exchange is to give you the big components of what is in my head. To start, creating and identifying safe spaces to be vulnerable is key. There is a book related to this that I would recommend entitled *Daring Greatly* by Dr. Brené Brown. Her book discusses shame and vulnerability backed up by tons of data she compiled and analyzed over the years. She defines the terms in distinct ways. A few quotes I want to bring up here:

> I define vulnerability as uncertainty, risk, and emotional exposure. (pg.34)

> Vulnerability is based on mutuality and requires boundaries and trust. It's not oversharing...Vulnerability is about sharing our feelings and our experiences with people who have earned the right to hear them. (pg. 46)

Shame is the intensely painful feeling
or experience of believing that we are
flawed and therefore unworthy of love
and belonging. (pg. 69)

Dr. Brown also discusses the "never-enough
problem" and terms people that have come to the
realization they are enough as the "wholehearted". I
read this book late in the game, yet it linked a lot of
other pieces of the mystery and gave me a better way
of describing my process in a way that could make it
practical and applicable to others.

One more reference before I walk you through
this first piece on safe spaces, and it is Matthew 13: 3-
9:

> 3 Then he told them many things in
> parables, saying: "A farmer went out
> to sow his seed. 4 As he was scattering
> the seed, some fell along the path, and
> the birds came and ate it up. 5 Some
> fell on rocky places, where it did not
> have much soil. It sprang up quickly,
> because the soil was shallow. 6 But
> when the sun came up, the plants
> were scorched, and they withered
> because they had no root. 7 Other
> seed fell among thorns, which grew up
> and choked the plants. 8 Still other
> seed fell on good soil, where it
> produced a crop—a hundred, sixty or
> thirty times what was sown. 9
> Whoever has ears, let them hear."

This verse is important to me because it is describing the differences between knowledge, understanding, and wisdom. An article entitled "You Don't Know What You Don't Know: Knowledge, Understanding, and Wisdom"[1] describes the three so succinctly. Knowledge is the facts, the data, the information, in its purest form. Understanding is getting what the facts mean and what are the values and principles that underlie those facts. Wisdom is application and knowing how to use the facts in context. Wisdom is the good soil in the parable. Wisdom is getting "it", getting life. I concede that without vulnerability, you cannot have wisdom. Without getting that we are enough, we have unproductive and unfulfilling lives starving for something we desire.

The reason I am promoting safe spaces to be vulnerable is it fosters and nurtures our soil so that when facts come our way, we can understand and then know what to do with them. I believe you need multiple safe spaces because the more vulnerable you can be among diverse perspectives, the more likely you can sort out what is true and what is not, what is you and what is not. If you find that you are trying to grow with only you and maybe with a couple of inputs from a few people, it is danger sign. We are a community and thrive in community. If we are to grow, we must connect ourselves with as much community that is representative of humanity as possible. Our greatest minds and souls that have walked this earth, our sages, knew this. That is why

[1] https://tifwe.org/you-dont-know-what-you-dont-know-knowledge-understanding-and-wisdom

we find letters and other communications across cultural divides. Each person you engage tests your vulnerabilities and your assumptions. It is crazy uncomfortable yet exhilarating.

Knowledge builds on itself and often comes in unexpected ways. Starting from the break-up, the resources I needed to realize my truth came in constant flow, including specific safe spaces for me. Some already existed like parents, my closest friend Shawni Richardson (https://www.shawnirichardson.com), my other close family and friends, my community group through the Lower Manhattan Community Church (LMCC, http://www.lowermanhattanchurch.com/), and professional therapy sessions. Others were new such as a self-improvement group that focused on limitations and my coach Diazina Mobley (http://www.mindfulguidancesolutions.com/).

These new spaces were unconventional for me and required significant financial investment. In the title of the article I reference above on knowledge, understanding, and wisdom, the phrase appears "you don't know what you don't know." There are people, communities and formal organizations that have practiced and applied certain principles and truths with good results. In my circumstance, an invisible ceiling and barrier existed that I could not figure out how to break through. A frustration pervaded my every day because I possessed all these dreams, goals, and desires. I achieved a great deal so far and felt blessed for sure; but true wealth in life, the sense of fullness and ability to affect more than oneself, was missing.

I am not saying you have to try what I tried or

what I found value in. The key is to identify and frame your question that indicates what do you want to see more of and where do you think you are not getting it in life. Once your question is out there, let your eyes and ears be receptive and observant. Who or what is trying to answer your question, what type of data do they already have, and what type of results have they experienced first-hand? Sometimes it is worth just trying something even if you don't know if it will answer your question. Being willing to invest in myself and take risks on my growth opened me to tools, knowledge, and methods that I would not have gotten on my own. If our circles in life aren't expanding and shifting, the greater risk is stagnation.

Hey, it is apparent you want the best life and you want to reach your furthest dream. You are not ok with where you are but you may not know how to change it to be any different. I guarantee that the more safe spaces you cultivate in your life and the more you invest in you, the more you will shoot through the limitations in your life and grow and produce exponentially.

The benefits of safe spaces to be vulnerable for me were: 1) I humanized me and began to appreciate and accept the present me which is all that ever exists 2) I humanized others and moved away from people as a means or a barrier to my desires 3) I learned ways of interacting and exploring the world that made it a more enjoyable and richer journey with less stress and expectations 4) I became empowered to move through fear and "be" and 5) I am no longer lost, blind and deaf in the world-- my soil is fertile.

5 THE WAR

So I've given you my premise on safe spaces. It is a good time to discuss the war. Being able to humanize people including ourselves brings home the message in the scripture Ephesians 6:12 which states "For we wrestle not against flesh and blood..." Every atrocity and evil to rear its head in time starts with a lie. There are so many shapes the lie takes and the number of terms for it are vast. Check out Wikipedia: https://en.wikipedia.org/wiki/Lie. They list thirty-six terms. To give just a sample: Bad faith, Barefaced lie, Big lie, Bluffing, Cover-up, Deception, Defamation, Deflecting, Disinformation, Fabrication, Fake news, Fib, Fraud, Half-truth, Honest lie, Perjury, Speaking with forked tongue, White lie.

The lie is the source of the fall of humans from the beginning until present day. It comes from the east, west, north, south; it comes from our inner and outer being; and it appears out of thin air. Lies are like no-see-ums, biting flies. Some are only annoying while others can cause grave disease. Lies were set up by the darkness which the Bible names Satan and others find other names for destruction. Why does Satan and darkness exist? There is a supernatural dynamic that I won't fully understand while on this earth—maybe the answer will be revealed in eternity. What I must recognize is that Satan and darkness exist. The reason I must recognize this is because I found when I did not acknowledge a lie, it passed itself off as truth. It also passed itself off as part of me. It is like looking at a leech on your arm and saying it is a skin mole. Those moles begin to look like holes.

That is the genius of the lie—to make us see and believe what does not exist or to ignore what does exist. It is the fantasy generator and it can do so with only words. That is why the words we use and the words we embrace are so important. Words are the most powerful weapon on both sides of light and darkness. The words of darkness are always lies.

My theory is the two biggest aims of lies are to get you to believe: 1) you have holes meaning you are missing something, you are not enough, you need something to make you complete and 2) you are different in different areas of your life and you can compartmentalize your life into neat boxes. These two results bring you to a place of instability and confusion because aim #1 flays the perception of control from you and aim #2 reinforces the perception of control so with the two in action you are tossed to and fro (Ephesian 4:14).

Aim #1 comes up in many of the resources and programs I mentioned, so this is well known and in plain sight; yet, I don't know anyone that doesn't struggle with a feeling of being incomplete or wrong at least at some if not many points in their life. The

Bible says we lack nothing (Psalm 34:10). If you look at psychology, philosophies, and religious and spiritual practices, similar words abound. We are whole and completely human all the time. If I lose a leg or arm in battle, I am still human fully and completely. If I commit a crime, I am still human fully and completely. If I find myself enslaved, I am still fully and completely human. If I am poor and have no money, I am still fully and completely human. If I can't have a child from my womb, I am still fully and completely human. If I fail miserably and lose every possession and relationship I have, I am still fully and completely human. Nothing will change my DNA to say anything else. Even when you look at Sci-Fi, and mutants if that is even feasible, it is really enhancing the human, adding on not taking away. There is such perfection in humanity. We are each invaluable works of living art with our complete set of unique characteristics on all levels—spirit, soul, mind, and body.

Now Aim #2 is set up to prevent the absorption of words of truth, it is trying, very successfully, to rob us of wisdom which is the treasure we need to seek. "How much better to get wisdom than gold, to get insight rather than silver!" (Proverbs 16:16) I am all of me wherever I go even as I engage in a variety of activities, make several changes to what I do and how I do it, and interact with different individuals and groups. This means whenever I say I am working on one area of my life, I am working on all areas. This was apparent when I was working on self-development goals like pursuing writing or becoming more healthy.

To understand this, the pursuit of education and

career success has come with relative ease while romantic relationships have not. These two boxes in my life felt so disconnected. In my safe spaces, I came to acquire a large amount of knowledge and understanding with the awareness that as I began to grow and make progress towards improving my record on romantic relationships, it exposed relationships across my life, including in the artificial career box, in a way that showed where I could increase my vulnerability, express more of me, and show up more fully and humanely. If I did not embrace the truth that there are no boxes, I would think about what I learned as only to be used when it comes to entering and maintaining a romantic relationship losing the power of the data and cutting my productivity and ability to grow a crop of relationships in abundance.

We can't take advantage of the value of wisdom when we accept the lies aimed at compartmentalizing our existence. It is like having a full bank account and believing you can only use your bank card in one or two stores. You allow an artificial limit on your life.

The reason for presenting these aims of lies is not for awareness only. The insight I acquired over the last year or so (the insight blowing my mind) is the insight that can directly counteract the aims of lies and if applied could be what we need to spring forth. If we can work together to turn this understanding into true wisdom in mass, we can began producing a harvest of good and truth that will overtake the craziness and hate wreaking havoc in our societies without force and violence on our part. This section is a warning and an admonishment to put your watchdog goggles on for the true enemy because the more you get close to truth and wisdom, the attack of lies will come in an onslaught. Even as I am writing this to you, there is a battle waging in me saying stop and saying this is not worth writing. I fight every minute to keep going, not sure if this is a rehash or will ever be seriously taken by anyone.

These thoughts going through me are lies. The worst thing you can do is ignore lies. Don't ignore. Diazina talked to me about the dangers of not acknowledging the thoughts and voices that come into our heads. To ignore them gives them more power and motivation to keep going. To acknowledge them is not to say they are yours. That is a big point for me--not every thought that comes into my head is me. Many of them are not me and many of them are lies. To acknowledge them is to say to them "I see you." Once exposed, I can evaluate them against what I know and what I value as good. If they do not align, then they are kicked out and labeled as not mine.

On a related yet side note, rushing and lack of choice are lies. If you ever feel you have no choice or you feel forced or rushed, you are under the bondage of lies. That I know with all certainty in my being. These are flares saying "help me." When you are overwhelmed in this regard, do all you can to stand on what you know and seek out trusted loved ones and your safe spaces to douse you in truth such that you can free yourself. It is much quoted for a reason: "Then you will know the truth, and the truth will set you free." (John 8:32).

6 BE STILL

Before I go further into the core of my treatise, it is crucial for me to go over the safest space to be vulnerable which I alluded to somewhat. The safest place is a place of prayer and meditation. It is the place where you build moments with God. We are spiritual beings and when we ignore this fact, we do ourselves a great disservice and make life more difficult than it needs to be. When I with complete presence of mind go into an expectant place where I anticipate communing with the divine, there is always a response. Now, I may not always trust the response, and the response may not make sense, but there is a response. God's presence is felt, experienced, heard, and real when and only when we are present—when our spirit, soul, mind and body are in the now. Answers and provision come only in the now. If you find your thought and emotional energy are focused in the past or in the future, pause and reposition yourself to return to now. There are few guarantees that I would stake my life. One I mentioned and the other is this—everything that you need in any given moment including God is in the now. The scripture "Be still and know that I am God" (Psalm 46:10) embodies this guarantee. Did you know the meaning of the word "still" is more than not moving and making a sound. The definitions I pulled into my journal from different dictionary sources on the web:

> #1—not exerting; not moving a muscle; not trying to make things happen; calm, peace; not trying to make moves and set things in motion

> #2—even now; be in the now; be in the present; up to this time, but don't try to go any further

The definitions, especially in #2, hit me. With eight words, the Bible sums up our to-do-list and our jobs as humans. We are to live in the now, being at peace, not forcing life and standing on faith and allowing God be the "I am", allowing the desires of our heart to manifest in our lives.

I am going to recount to you a story my cousin told me that emphasizes this point well. She, her sister, and brother were working one weekend on renovations on a fixer-upper for her brother's family. They went to a second hand shop to scout out materials they could use. They set all six of their eyes on an amazing solid wood staircase. They desired it for they saw it would be perfect for the new house. This staircase had to be a ridiculous cost—so they thought. Could they afford it? Even if they could, how to get a 500lb wooden structure to where they wanted it to go? Instead of giving up the idea, they started with asking the price. The man said "$400." This was too much and not within the brother's budget. They asked again and the man said he could let it go for $280. That price the brother could accept. He happened to have a dump truck he was using that could fit the staircase. They went to go get it and returned to the store. At first it looked like they would have to get it in the truck on their own but then men working nearby said they could use their forklift to help my cousins. So the staircase made it on the truck and my cousins returned to the house. At the house, they did not have a forklift so how were the three of them, made of two petite ladies and a pretty lean guy, get their prize into this house. The first step was getting it off the truck. They decided to try. Low and behold the staircase made it off the truck still intact. Ok, now how were they going to get it through the door and in position inside the house? The cousins looked at each other and said let's give it a try. I think you know the ending—they got the beautiful staircase into the house and in position. This amazed my cousin telling me the story. This fit so nicely in to our discussion around my insight regarding a richer life.

This showed if you reach out in the moment for what you need and want, the provision or answer for it is there even if it doesn't make sense or you can't immediately figure out the full steps or plan of action. If we can take just one action and one step, that is all it takes. The old folks knew this, that is why they always used to say "I'm just taking it one day at a time."

As a human being, you do not have the capacity to do more than that. If you try, you will fall flat on your face because you are trying to be what you are not. You are not God. You are not the universe. You are not above time or space. To want or believe you are more than what you are is the recipe for the fall of man. I see this repeating pattern in my own life. I sought to figure out the future and force its hand and it led to my biggest failures and showed my immense fallibility. This is not to say one will not make mistakes or fail if you are in the now. Because we are growing and learning, we haven't reached the full pinnacle of who we are and may not before our death. What I believe it will do is make the time here on earth the most productive and beautiful and rich time ever, not only for you, but also for everyone with whom you interact and connect.

Let me step back because I don't want to preach to you for this is supposed to be a proposal, a topic to be discussed and hashed out between us. I get so riled up about observing the secularization of society on so many levels. It is not about religion. It is about the working of the human being. As individuals, how can we choose to dismiss or not utilize a critical component of our operation. Too often we go straight to our thoughts, our logic, then to our emotions, that sets off our actions. The spirit is where the roots ground us and the seeds of creativity germinate. The spirit feeds our heart, the seat of our desires. The spirit tells us what is possible. It holds the knowing and the mysteries of the universe. It activates our desires, our dreams. To ignore the spirit is to only seek cut flowers and not the full plant. The cut flowers will have beauty for a time and give you some joy in their existence but it is short-lived and you can't get more from what you have. Once it is wilted and dried, it is gone. If you appreciate the full plant and seek it, you get seasons and life cycles of fruit and flowers and the possibility of expanding your garden to have more of the same.

The intentional accessing of the spirit at as many conscious moments as possible will help us combat lies, be more vulnerable and therefore more human, and manifest the truth of life in a more powerful way equaling wisdom. As I have pursued knowledge and resources in different places whether through the programs listed, books, and even movies, there are similar principles that I believe are universal truths yet employed in secular contexts.

It came together for me while watching the movie The Secret about the law of attraction. I had not read the book but heard about it numerous times for years and dismissed it as fluff and too much like the ineffective name-it-and-claim-it movement. It seemed to me a misrepresentation of positive thinking or so I thought. These conclusions were made even though I had not taken the time to figure out what it was saying. After watching the movie, I was floored. It was like a string of lights illuminating in progression.

In summary, the movie and the different coaching and personal growth resources in my life at the time indicated that wanting is what humans do and what we want is possible. To see what we want manifested in the world, we have to focus on what you want to see in the world, and wherever your energy is focused, that is where you produce fruit and where you see manifestation. Basically, you identify a desire, visualize with all senses that desire, know it is there and exists, and allow it to come and manifest in its time. This sounded familiar to me. It was what the Bible indicates as faith. "Now faith is the substance of things hoped for, the evidence of things not seen." (Hebrews 11:1) God was telling us this truth all along. I believe we see people accessing this truth all the time and we term them the haves. I think they do it in a secular way there manifesting temporary or counterproductive results, yet truth is truth so will be effective even if employed in a partial way. Maybe that is why you have many that do not believe in God tithe, give a portion of their wealth away, because they recognize the truth of the exercise.

It still bothered me that I was understanding faith more than ever and was getting the concept, yet wasn't seeing a consistent application or result in my own life. My strong gut tugged within me and said if there was a way to tie spirit to a truth that was operating in the secular, it would manifest with more power and explode on impact in a positive way. If I and as many others, especially who I consider missing in this imbalance world, could translate truth to wisdom, it would be the healing and salvation we need. We would show up whole and connected--the new Eden.

One key message in the movie The Secret that stuck with me most was this idea of focusing on what you want to see in the world versus what you don't want to see. What you focus on is what you will see. One of the speakers in the film gave the example of debt and how people say they want to get out of debt or want to be debt free. He said "you are still thinking about debt." The key was focusing on what you want which is to have enough, to be prosperous, to be financially secure. A modern day example of this principle is the 2016 United States elections. I believe, and read a couple of articles along these lines, because the media and the country focused so much on Donald Trump and fighting against him to prevent his presidency, they got exactly what they did not want. There was little energy going into putting forward and investing in building what they wanted in a president. We can continue this more global view and application of truth later. It is important that we first get more understanding on a personal level.

7 AHA! MOMENT

I am really close to the "aha!" moment, the big bang. Here is one more story to set it up. One of the greatest blessings in my life is the extent to which I have been able to travel and experience other cultures through my career. One trip was to Italy for a conference in Tuscany. The conference was 5 days and I decided and planned my flights to have 4 days in Rome. For the months preceding, I was learning more and more this idea of the law of attraction and faith, and I tried to exercise it as much as I could. The trip presented an opportunity. The opportunity to put out there what I wanted and see it manifested. For the trip, I wanted to have the conference and side meeting that I had a part in organizing to be a success, to have a wonderful place in Rome to stay, to see key sights I had identified, to fit in a visit to Florence, to go to the beach, and to have a male companion of some sort to be able to share the experiences. After the trip, I recapped my trip to Diazina indicating all the amazing manifestations on the trip. I experienced everything that I wanted except for the companion. It was wonderful and exciting to see evidence of the principle in a real and personal way. What nagged at me was the one request that was not granted. Why? Diazina said that because I had resistance in the area of relationships, this area was slower to manifest and I would not see results so quickly. The word "resistance" stuck out for me. What is resistance? To me, I allowed in the moment for a companion; I was sure of it. Remember, romantic relationships and relationships with men are to me my weakest and most challenging area of life. I have definitely grown in understanding of intimacy and relationship with men which involves a deeper relationship to self so felt tons of progress, yet..

Diazina lovingly explained resistance to me. Resistance, she said, is a quality within us that arises in areas of our life where we feel lack. It already came to my attention that any lack on my part is perceived lack because as a human being I am whole and complete lacking nothing. She further advised me to explore and look at any area of my life where I felt lack and where I didn't see manifestation of my desires. The other requests and desires for my Italy trip came to be because if they manifested or didn't, my trip would have still been great. I did not feel one way or the other if they happened or not. Those requests were not filling any holes. With having a companion, I felt the tinge of emotion and even though I called my trip a success, the lack of an obvious companion bothered me. I say obvious because during the conference, the beach trip especially, I was surrounded by new friends and people to share my experience. In some ways, I was not alone, I just didn't recognize it as satisfying my request.

I share the Italy trip for this reason; after my session with Diazina, I sat on my couch after church on a Sunday holding my Bible and asking for some word from God. Personal growth is a consistent discomfort. This particular Sunday, the discomfort pressed me hard. I sat there to get to my ok and truth space. The word "treasure" came to me. I googled "treasure scriptures". A few scripture were listed and scanned them and picked two. It was my recent practice to read the full chapter of the verse. The first and only chapter I begin to read, Matthew 13, came to the forefront. I have already recounted the first 9 verses. The following verses are what ignited my fire and had me jumping for joy. I called Shawni and bounced this insight off of her. I then began meeting up for lunch and dinner with other friends and doing the same. It is the "aha!" for me, the key we need to get the truth of life.

> 10 And the disciples came, and said unto him, Why speakest thou unto them in parables? 11 He answered and said unto them, Because it is given unto you to know the mysteries of the kingdom of heaven, but to them it is not given. 12 For whosoever hath, to him shall be given, and he shall have more abundance: but whosoever hath not, from him shall be taken away even that he hath.

If we lack nothing, are wholehearted, and are

complete, then if we have not it is because we have a perceived deficiency or lack that we cannot see how to overcome. One women's program I joined explored what it means to be a woman and working to express more of the essence of women in this world. In talking with women about the program, we often ask them two questions and you can ask yourself this as well: 1) what do you want? 2) why do you want it?

Underlying every desire we have is a deeper desire or perceived need. What do we think that specific desire will give us or add to us. If we can identify the underlying perceived lack, we then take the next step of looking at our life and working to recognize where we have what we think we are missing. The problem with perceived lack is that it does not exist, we are chasing a vapor. Our pursuit becomes more about the chase then the actual item we are reaching for. We are not be able to recognize our desire even if it slapped us in the face.

Someone mentioned something similar to me as I was pursuing a goal around dating. I didn't get his point fully at the time and now I do. This perceived lack is why we see someone in our lives seeking relationships or specific response from people that seem opposite to what they say they want and then reject others in their life that are giving them what they say they want. A very close familiar relationship was like that for me. I felt I was giving this person so much in love and respect, yet what I was doing was never enough and they continued to complain that I did not love or respect them. This hurt me, but now I see the person had a huge perceived hole in their being that could not be filled because it did not exist.

This awareness of perceived lack and the underlying desires we have is so important. It is this awareness we can use to examine our life as a whole and take our appreciation and gratitude lists, the ones that are on trend for a reason. If we can find where we have in our lives, we will with ease have more. The secular world uses this mostly in material and temporal ways. How more amazing it would be to use not only in material and temporal ways, but in value-based and principled ways to build and produce more love, peace, and respect in this world.

A couple of days after that Sunday of insight, I went to lunch with a friend of mine, that I had not seen for at least a year. Her recent life events illustrated my points so well. She revealed that she recently near the beginning of the summer broke off a relationship. The pain and grief of it really got her down. It was a bad break-up. She had been the type of person front and center of the happenings in New York City especially during the summer. This event in her life drove her into a place of isolation. She said another friend of hers told her to find her place of love. She thought about it and decided to get off her fanny and take a friend up on her invitation to visit her family in the Mid-West. She went and enjoyed thoroughly hanging out with the friend and her two young children. It lifted her heart and she returned to NYC more invigorated, yet still sad. Then, her family from down south, over 40 of them, decided to come up the east coast to the nation's capital, and she went down to meet them. It was the most joyful experience; I witnessed it through her social media feed. She said to me that after those two trips she felt so loved and so encouraged. She then had 48 hours in the city before she was to go take some time for self-love for a week or two at an apartment about two hours out of town belonging to a friend who was going on a long trip abroad. During that 48-hour period, another friend contacted her to have drinks and feeling in a better place and wanting to see this friend she agreed. At the lounge where they met, the bartender, who also had other interesting side gigs like many New Yorkers, took a liking to her and they exchanged numbers. The two have been talking ever since. She commented that it was so nice to be connected with him because of the love and respect he shows to her. She didn't think about the future trying to make it more than what it was at that moment, just appreciating it for what it was. I believe that because she actively went into her life and found the places where she felt love and acceptance, it opened the door for her to get more of it from unexpected places (i.e., meeting the bartender).

Shawni sent me an excerpt that further speaks to this from the Armor of God Devotional by Pricilla Striner:

> Paul wasn't asking in prayer that the Ephesian believers would receive their abundant inheritance of spiritual riches, blessings, power, and authority, but that they would realize it was theirs. As Christians, they already possessed these things, just as we do. But until they realized it, what good could it accomplish?
>
> In reality, the spiritual armor he describes in Ephesians 6 is merely a

repeat of—a different way of describing—what Paul had been explaining in the first portion of the letter. How could they "put on" or "take up" things they didn't know they had? The first step for them—the first step for us—in utilizing the spiritual resources we've been given is to have our spiritual eyes opened so that we can see them.

The story of Elisha and his vision-impaired servant in 2 Kings 6 is one of my absolute favorite stories in the Bible. The setting is a battle about to ensue between the enraged king of Aram and the nation of Israel.

Elisha's servant got an eyeful. At first, he could only see the enemy, which likely left him no other response than fear and anxiety.

But then he immediately became tuned in to a game-changing spiritual reality: more was at his disposal and working on his behalf than he could have ever imagined. What his physical eyes could see were no match for what they couldn't see. Elisha's prayer helped make him aware of all the resources and strength on his side fighting against the enemy.

To be confident and victorious, you've got to be able to "see" it.

In Ephesians 1, Paul accentuates just a few of the gifts God has given us. There are many more, and each one connects specifically with your spiritual armor and weapons. The first key to understanding how they all fit into your ability to pin down the enemy is vision. You cannot use them if you're not able to fully recognize them, if you're not aware of their availability and their importance in successfully waging war against the enemy.

If we can practice and apply this "having" and "no lack" truth into our lives, it will shift and transform us amazing ways. One of the ultimate results of the lies and the instability of the two aims of lies is a life drowning in fear. David in Psalm 64 cried "Hear my voice, O God, in my prayer: preserve my life from fear of the enemy." It is not the unseen enemy that will destroy us, it is the fear of that enemy that will destroy us. The darkness does not have to lift a finger. Fear is the fruit of lies. Fear has consumed us so badly that we are afraid of existing because we are afraid we are getting it wrong. There is nothing we are getting wrong. I attended an annual church retreat at LMCC and the guest speaker, Pastor Drew Hyun, ended the retreat with the following words:

We are all...
Fully Loved
Fully Accepted
...and we have...
Nothing to Hide
Nothing to Prove
Nothing to Fear

8 JOIN ME

Can you see why I am so excited? The effects of
oppression and enslavement are evident in the lives of
women across the globe, and really among all human
beings. We are objectified and dehumanized beyond
measure. It is up to us to stand fully in our humanity
and show up. If we focus on attaining a unshakable
knowing that we are a human being lacking *nothing*,
our very presence will cause change. My desire is that
you will take up this challenge with me to practice and
work daily to apply this truth from a desire as small as
choosing something to buy to an event to as big as
world peace. We are adept at community and building
and connecting with human beings in every corner of
the earth. Can you imagine walking into an
environment and by being who you are, the principles
you want to see are manifested?

Because we are the offspring and children of God,
I believe the "why we are here" is to create and build
as crazily and as exceptionally as our hearts desire. I
believe earth is our playground and that it grieves

God that we don't see it as such. I also believe Jesus came to restore the original plan. We are to play together and connect and go wild. There are no boundaries on any plane, so hand in hand with you, I want to break free and be. With love.

ABOUT THE AUTHOR

Dr. C. P. Scott is a humanitarian and global health specialist. She has dedicated her personal and professional life to working towards and scaling solutions for impoverished communities. Her vision is to contribute to the advancement and empowerment of women, specifically women of color. Dr. Scott received her Ph.D. in International Health from Johns Hopkins University. She has a Master of Public Health (MPH) degree and B.S. in Biology from Florida A & M University.